Walk of
HOPE

One Woman's Journey with Multiple Sclerosis

Christine Ganger

Outskirts Press, Inc.
http://www.outskirtspress.com

ISBN: 978-1-4787-7536-2

Outskirts Press and the "OP" logo are trademarks belonging to Outskirts Press, Inc.

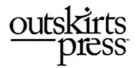

PRINTED IN THE UNITED STATES OF AMERICA

What others are saying about this book:

Cont. from cover ...

Christine is a pure inspiration. She is one of the strongest women I know. Through her story, you will read about the difficult situations she faces with her M.S. Yet every day with God's help she finds the positive in everything! She is always trying to help people through her experience and listen to the voice of God.

Walk of Hope is a perfect title for this book! It will give you the strength and the hope to never give up! Christine is real and honest about her battle with M.S.

-Shelley Green

───────────────

Christine has given her readers a true gift of authentic living. She bravely reveals her shattered dreams, fractured relationships, wavering faith, heartbreaking decisions and sorrows of the heart. Through her life story, you will discover a woman who is resolute in heart, soul and mind; she refuses to cave into life woes and courageously hopes in God, knowing He has purpose for her life. She intends to live her life with vigor and love, knowing God has chosen her to impact lives for Him.

-Robyn L. Crowley
Founder/CEO Women's Growth Institute

Walk of Hope

A Woman's Journey with Multiple Sclerosis

Christine Ganger

Cassopolis, Michigan

Copy Edited by Jeanie Correa

For
Royann Cross

I dedicate this book to my friend and confidant, Royann Cross. I wish I could have finished this story prior to her sudden death so we could have read it together.

Royann was an incredible friend. It is a special privilege to have a friend one can trust unconditionally—to share my inner most thoughts and feelings. Royann helped me to better understand myself and recognize the best in myself. She was the wisest woman I ever knew, and she made *me* a wiser person, as well.

I will miss our times together, Royann, but I will always treasure the memories and apply the lessons I learned from you.

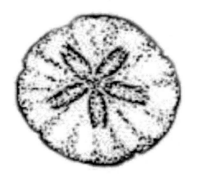

Table Of Contents

Table of Contents (Continued)

Table of Contents (Continued)

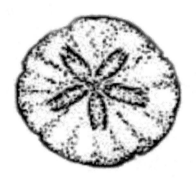

About the Author

Christine Ganger is an educator and freelance author. With a B.S in Elementary Education from Liberty University and an M.S. in Special Education from Indiana University, Christine has invested 20 years in the classroom, teaching and encouraging students to read and write. It is her life's desire to love and encourage others, as evidenced by a nomination for Teacher of the Year, winner of Most Creative Teacher award, and countless lives that have been impacted.

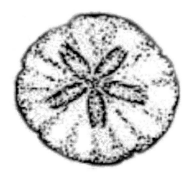

Acknowledgement

I would like to acknowledge my friend, Robyn Crowley. She believed God was writing a story for me to share. She helped and encouraged me through the entire process. God bless you, my friend!

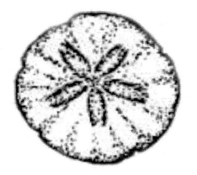

INTRODUCTION

We are all fighting a battle. My daily battle is Multiple Sclerosis (MS). My desire is that somehow my story will inspire in you the courage to choose hope each day, whatever your battle or challenge might be.

About MS

Multiple sclerosis is a disease that affects the central nervous system; and more specifically, the immune system directly attacks the brain and spinal cord. It can cause problems of varying severity with muscle control and strength, vision, balance, feeling, and thinking.

The exact cause is unknown. There is no cure for MS.

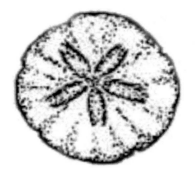

Chapter One

My Early Days

I was an unplanned pregnancy—the first of two daughters—a little detail that my parents would not reveal until after they were properly married and living officially as husband and wife.

In my young life I was quite the tomboy, dividing my time between camping, Girl Scouts, climbing trees and playing Little League.

As a child, God was not a subject of conversation in our household; and had that remained so, I might have never known about faith and what it would allow me to accomplish as I faced a world of obstacles. But that would all change when I entered the fourth grade.

Loneliness befell my mother as the family settled into our new home in our new neighborhood, as dad worked 12-hour nights—when he wasn't out of town, that is. To fill her time, she found a Christian radio station that would one day change the trajectory of generations to come.

A late-night Christian radio program called Night Sounds broadcast throughout the house that fateful night as mom dutifully went about washing and scrubbing down the kitchen walls. She had already taken to reading the Bible, as a result of her new Christian radio hobby bringing her the message of hope 24/7. And before she knew it, before the clock struck the midnight hour, before it was too late, my mom gave her heart, and her family, over to Jesus.

Her salvation experience would take another 10 years to impact my father, and in the interim the atmosphere at home was consistently tense. In her zeal to do right by God, her nudging was often misconstrued as nagging by a husband who wasn't ready to give up the grand illusions of drinking and gambling.

That same year, mom went to work at a Christian school as the lunch lady. And within a year, she had arranged to have me transferred over to the same school. Resentful and resistant, I wanted nothing to do with it and especially hated the thought of wearing a dress to school every day. But my mom's diligence, as well as the constant feeding of God's Word at my new school, eventually paid off on my eternity. At age 11, I came to know Jesus as my savior.

I can't say that my life appeared to change as a result; but in retrospect, I'm confident God put a hedge of protection around my future, beginning at that moment in time. I attended Christian school from fifth grade on.

Chapter Two

High School

I found myself transferring schools yet again as my school was closing its doors for good. In spite of being reassigned to my rival school, I transitioned nicely and had four wonderful years of high school.

Prior to high school, I had been relatively shy. For the most part I was pretty easy going, but I had my moments. Whenever I got upset, I would go to the batting cage and take my frustration out on the balls. Then a shift happened as I finished up my eighth grade. As I gave myself completely to school sports and cheerleading, I quickly came out of my shell. I was a good kid through high school, had friends and enjoyed just being. I think being involved in sports, working, and dating good guys helped me stay out of trouble. I even had a job. I was happy—and healthy.

Much of my future was shaped in my junior and senior year, as I spent many a study hall periods helping in the Learning Disabled (LD) classroom. I flip-flopped over college degree and career choices that I felt needed to be answered now. I took aptitude tests to point me in a logical direction, but the options just made it harder. From forest ranger to travel guide to teacher, the possibilities were like night and day. I had always liked adventure and the outdoors. My future seriously would come down to choosing between outdoor wildlife or classroom wildlife! I knew helping kids felt good. Since I had never been a great student and studies weren't always easy for me, I thought I could be understanding and perhaps help others. Besides, the outdoors was something I'd have the rest of my life to enjoy after work and on weekends, right?

With a friend's help I realized that, ultimately, what I wanted to do was teach. When I told my mom this was my plan, she laughed, reminding me of a childhood proclamation I had made in response to an elementary teacher saying, "I don't want to be a teacher when I grow up; I want people to like me." And so it turned out that I would become an LD teacher.

With Christian school education came lots of Bible learning. Though it seemed at times little more than useless head knowledge, I would live and grow to appreciate the jewels I worked so hard at taking to memory and hiding in my heart. Some would take years of living life to fully realize, but one verse in particular took root early on and would become my "life verse."

"Being confident of this very thing, that He who began a good work in you will carry it on to completion until the day of Christ Jesus."

~Philippians 1:6 NIV

To this day, I still call upon this scripture and make it my own; it has carried me through many dark places.

Chapter Three

Off to College

I wanted to go away to college, my dad said I needed to stay home and attend a local Indiana University extension to prove I would work and make decent grades. So I stayed home my freshmen year, working part time at an RV company imputing data and at the mall on evenings and weekends. I also coached cheerleading at my former high school. I kept pretty busy. In an introduction to teaching class, a professor told me, "perhaps you should think about a different major; teaching might not be for you." I wasn't completely certain why he felt this way, although I had a feeling it might have been prompted by my poor public speaking ability. I was determined, however, and I chose to continue the journey.

Dad's plan worked; I stayed home and my grades were good. And I wasn't a lazy freeloading college brat! But I so wanted to go away to school—Liberty University, to be exact. It was a big Christian school that had just become a university. My plan was to meet me a good ol' southern boy, get married and move out west to the mountains—bye bye, Midwest!

I got my wish the following fall, in 1988, and headed to Lynchburg, Virginia, to attend LU. My roommate was a friend of mine from high school. I loved it. I played intramurals and made lots of friends. In October, my friends even threw a surprise 21st birthday party for me at Chucky Cheese.

I managed to keep my grades up, which pleased my parents; but even better, I absolutely loved college life.

Chapter Four

First Signs of Illness

I spent that first Christmas break back home with my family and hanging with lots of high school friends. It was a wonderful time. I found myself getting these odd sensations—a dull pain behind my eye.

"I feel like I have a headache in my eye," I said on more than one occasion and was met with eye-rolling. I suppose it sounded somewhat silly to those not experiencing it. But I was used to getting headaches, so I did what I would normally do and took some ibuprofen, which seemed to help.

My roommate and I decided to take a modular course before the semester began. A modular course consists of going to class from 8 a.m. to 3 p.m. for five days to get three credits quickly.

Our drive to school took 12 hours. We left at 8 a.m. Saturday morning to get back and be ready for a Monday class. All the way up, I still had that darn headache in my eye. About three quarters of the way there, I told Cindy I wasn't seeing very well. She finished driving the last leg of the trip.

It was very quiet on campus. My head still hurt, but I thought it was just a migraine and that it would be better the next morning. No such luck.

I called my parents Sunday morning. The campus clinic was closed and I didn't have a doctor there. Mom and dad said to go ahead and go to the Emergency Room. By the time my roommate and I got to the ER, I couldn't see anything out of my right eye. The doctor in the emergency room asked me to read the eye chart.

"I know there is always an E on the top, but I sure can't see it," I told the doctor.

After a thorough examination, the doctor had no answers and suggested I go to an ophthalmologist. My hands were tied; I would have to wait till the following Monday, since nothing was open on Sunday.

Back at the dorm, my two roommates played doctor and the three of us experimented to see the reality of my vision loss. I would cover my left eye and they would toggle the lights off and on. It was affirmative; I could not see at all.

I went to class Monday morning. I explained to the professor what was going on and that I really wanted to complete the course. I was sure everything would be back to normal by the end of the week. He assured me it would be fine and we would do what we needed in order for me to complete the class.

I saw an ophthalmologist, but he urged me to see my family doctor. This seemed odd—he was an eye specialist. Why would he send me to a general practice doctor for an eye problem? I didn't have a family doctor there, and I had a class I was trying to finish.

My roommate was a real friend and trooper through the week. We spent all day in class, and then at night she would read the assignment aloud to me. Luckily the eye I could see out of was my strong eye. I could see just enough to write. And boy what a mess that was; my writing was large and sloppy. But I made it through the week, and I passed the course.

After a lot of expensive daily long distance phone calls home, my parents decided I should come home. And since I didn't have a car and I couldn't drive, my dad and a pastor friend from our church came and got me.

I finished my final exam Friday when dad showed up after a 12-hour drive only to turn around and drive right home.

I appeared fine when they saw me—a relief to my dad, I'm sure. I just wanted to get this over so I could get back for classes and to my friends.

The following Monday I saw the neurologist who, after an eye examination, reaffirmed his previous diagnosis of Optic Neuritis. The possibilities were that it could just go away on its own or it might be a precursor to Multiple Sclerosis. He ordered a spinal tap as a process of elimination.

As we waited for the spinal tap and my eyesight started to get better, my parents bought a plane ticket for the following Sunday night to get me back to school where I desperately wanted to be.

At the clinic, a nurse took me back to the examination room where I was met by a second nurse and a doctor. I spotted a syringe with what seemed a huge needle. The doctor explained the importance of lying very still for the procedure. He would be drawing some spinal fluid to test. In the fetal position and scared, both nurses held me so I didn't move. With the nurses constantly encouraging me, I managed to hold my breath and get beyond the needle and through the procedure just fine.

The rest of the day would prove to be quite deceiving as any indicator of how my next few months would go. Even though I was told I might experience a slight headache later, I was surprised at how good I felt. I still took their advice and took it easy for the rest of the day, lying around and watching T.V.

But the following morning things were not so good. As I showered, I quickly became sick to my stomach, until eventually vomiting.

"Mom," I summoned, and then back to bed for the rest of the day. Nausea persisted throughout the day, but I found that if

I lay flat on my back, I could keep it at bay for longer periods. What in the world is wrong with me, I wondered.

Sunday came, but instead of hopping a plane back to school, I was lying around home watching the super bowl and choking back tears. I wanted desperately to feel better and be back at school.

As it turned out, my spinal tap had been performed by an intern who failed to discharge me with the necessary after-care instructions. I should have laid flat for several hours following the procedure but was allowed to leave immediately.

The next few weeks crept. Nausea was the norm, and I felt terrible. And sad. I finally had to go back to Virginia with my parents and retrieve my belongings. It was a bittersweet trip; I was glad to see everyone, though I still couldn't stay up long without getting sick. But my dear friends decorated my old room and threw a get-well/going-away party for me.

While there, we attended a basketball game. Jerry Falwell walked by during the game and jokingly hit me in the back of the head.

"Jerry healed me," I would tell friends. I was so tired after the trip and time on campus, but I was especially sad to leave and head back home.

With the nausea improving each day, I discovered I needed something to fill my time to avoid boredom. I've never been good at doing nothing. Our church was in need of some part time help, so I jumped at it. I worked half days in the office running off bulletins and sending out mailings each week. I was happy to get out of the house and have something to do.

The following June I was feeling much better, allowing me to chaperone a junior high school group of girls on a wilderness trip to Canada through church. We canoed and then portaged our canoes to the next area and slept outside. The experience was incredible, and I was so thankful my health had improved enough to allow me this opportunity. I was feeling back to normal. I even played on a softball team that summer just as I had for the past several years. Surely this had all been a bad setback and would not progress further.

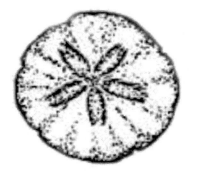

Chapter Five

More College, Progressive Illness

I spent my second college summer splitting my time between working at my church and at a boys and girls home, doing such tasks as reading and math tutoring, helping with dinner and tucking kids in at night.

I returned to Liberty as a junior, ready to tackle my third year. This time I had a boyfriend. But I was never able to reconnect to college life. I suppose that's the price one pays when spending what seems like every waking moment with her boyfriend. This made it difficult to connect with old friends or meet new ones. But it was more than that. My energy and strength were failing.

I completed the next two years; but just before starting the summer of 1991, I was painfully aware of my struggle to walk and maintain my balance. It had become extremely difficult to walk down to my classes from the dorm. At the end of my junior year, I started to lose my eyesight again. I now felt sure it was MS. And with my self-diagnosis, I decided that as an MS patient I would choose not to have children. If I couldn't be the mom I had always pictured, I would not be a mom at all.

On returning home for summer break, my doctor immediately sent me for an MRI. After the procedure, I would finally get the results we had all been dreading. It was a warm summer day and I recall sitting at the kitchen table when the phone rang. My dad answered. It was his friend, who also happened to be my family doctor.

"Hi," I heard him say in a flat voice. "What did you find out?" He fell silent for a moment.

"OK, what do we do now?"

I didn't have to ask. I knew the test had come back positive. Dad now faced me.

"The MRI shows lesions and it is MS," he said, choking back tears. "We need to get things together." He made us an appointment at an MS center in Chicago. He'd had a nurse who was diagnosed with MS and had gone to this same center. We were confident this was the best place for me to be.

"Pack a bag, just in case they want you to stay" he insisted.

"OK," I said and went to my room. I didn't want to be hugged or consoled. I was "just fine." We all went to our respective rooms, and my parents starting the process of making phone calls and informing friends and relatives of the diagnosis. This was very hard for them—and very emotional.

I cried from behind my bedroom door, though I would act like this was not a big deal. My packed bag consisted of a toothbrush and a pair of shorts. I couldn't imagine they would have me actually stay at the hospital.

With a new hospital, new doctor and even a nurse who herself had MS, we were confident this was the best place to be for us.

I rode with my parents to the hospital to find the MS Center. My doctor was a woman, and I really liked her. She had me perform various tests, which were far from easy. She had me walk in a straight line with one foot in front of the other, as well as stand with my eyes closed and my hands and arms out in front of me. I couldn't do it. I was frustrated and embarrassed. But I would be strong for my parents. They struggled so with the whole thing.

The doctor made it clear that there was currently no cure for MS, nor was there any medicine to treat it. Her team suggested I check in to the hospital for a 10-day massive ATCH steroid treatment. I was shocked.

I had never been in the hospital before. They sent us to the hospital cafeteria for lunch while a room was prepared for me. My nerves were now kicking in. I tried to act calm and continue like it was no big deal.

I would be given infusions for several hours every night. They put in a stint that would stay in my arm for a couple days until it needed replaced. I had to eat bland food so that my stomach didn't get upset. The only noticeable side effect was an uncomfortably puffy face.

The teaching staff sure got lucky with me; medical students could come in each day and examine and study me. I participated in physical therapy every day, strengthening my hips with exercises and some dance steps.

After the 10-day stay, my sight returned and I felt much stronger. But I was living in fear—fear of the future. In hindsight, I should never have made any major decisions, but I did. I got engaged to my boyfriend. It seemed like the right thing to do; he was a good guy. He loved me; and through a lifetime of taking care of his sick mother, it seemed he would know how to take care of me if it came to that. Friends since high school, we worked and played well together.

An interesting discovery through this visit was that heat can be very hard on people with MS. My home had always only had one window unit air conditioner in it, which happened to be in my parents' room. So after some studious research by my sister, Rona, mom and dad invested in whole-house central air and have enjoyed it ever since.

I was saddened by the diagnosis but didn't really believe it would progress. I think I chose to be optimistic and believe it would all be OK. What concerned me most was being treated differently because of the diagnosis. I wanted to be the same and wanted others to treat me the same.

The problem with that was I couldn't do all the things I did before. That was my reality; so, others stopped inviting me to activities in which I could no longer physically participate. Thoughtful, yes; but hurtful nonetheless.

After I was released from the hospital, my softball coach called to see if I wanted to play that summer. At my insistence that I could not run, he told me to come, play the field, and they would put a runner on for me if I just hit the ball and ran to first base. Discouraged, I went to the next game holding what little hope I had. Unfortunately, just playing catch before the came was all it took to make up my mind. Painfully aware of how big a problem my balance was, I knew there was no way I could play anymore.

I really didn't even know what kinds of things I could do that I would enjoy. I had always played sports, as did most of my friends. It was lonely, indeed. Ironically, some of that was my choice. I didn't want others to see or notice my difficulties: my walking was slow and unstable, I could no longer run nor walk long distances and I had become rather uncoordinated.

With my new physical limitations came a loss of confidence in many areas of my life. Sports had always been the language in which I was especially fluent—where my confidence lay.

Chapter Six

Graduation & Marriage

I was to do my student teaching in the fall to cmplete my Elementary Education degree. After the diagnosis, I contacted the University and I was able to complete my student teaching at an area elementary school. While I certainly wanted to complete my degree, at this point I wondered if I would ever teach. At least I had a wedding I could focus on.

I graduated in May 1992 and was married in July.

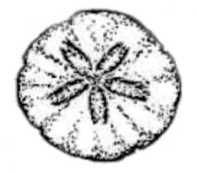

Chapter Seven

Teaching & Staggering

I started substitute teaching in the fall. This allowed me to work on my good days, and I felt good about actually getting some use out of my degree. The MS mostly affected my lower extremities, which wrecked my balance and left me weak. I'm sure I appeared drunk with my MS stagger, which grew even worse with fatigue. A perpetual numbness in my legs meant having to stretch them before I stood to walk.

Other issues were arising that I had to learn to deal with. I found myself having to use the bathroom often, but I could never seem to completely empty my bladder. And there was the matter of twitching in my legs, which made it hard to sleep. My solution was to take advantage of my flexibility and go to sleep with my legs crossed, Indian style, and lie over them. That little life hack got me to sleep, but if I woke up needing to go to the bathroom, there was a problem: my legs would be asleep from having cut off the circulation and I couldn't walk at all. Turns out, oddly, that the restless leg syndrome wasn't the fault of my MS after all, but an inherited condition that I would soon find I shared with both my mom and her mom.

In the fall of 1994 I checked back in to the hospital for yet another steroid stay, but this time would be for only five days.

By this time they were making a lot of progress with medicines and used a different type of steroid. And since the process was familiar to me, it wasn't nearly as scary this time around. The day I was released was actually my birthday, which was gift enough! The five-day treatment revitalized me, and my legs felt strong and ready to try to run. Of course that didn't turn out quite like I'd hoped. Regardless, I was just excited to feel like I could run again. That was enough—for now.

I was becoming stronger and more confident when, in the spring, I started a part-time paraprofessional position. I was hopeful that I could do this, and it would bring me one step closer to becoming a teacher. The following year a position opened in the LD room and I went full time.

I became a teacher in September of 1995. A first grade position opened after school had already begun. I poured myself into my teaching. In the meantime, I was determined to exercise my body each morning for 20 minutes before work. I discovered that getting my legs moving and loosened up helped set the pace for my workday. I used a stationary rider at home, which involved pushing with my legs and pulling with my arms.

My friends list dwindled, most having families of their own and leading busy lives. I got a shelter dog, Snickers, who was great company and loved me unconditionally. He filled the empty spot in my bed on Tom's work travel nights away, perpetually inching his head over to my pillow for a little snuggle time.

Chapter Eight

Popularity & Infidelity

Turns out I loved teaching and wanted more! People liked me and I was now making friends. No one knew, yet, about my MS. My students liked me, the parents seemed to like me and I got along wonderfully with the other teachers and administration.

With all the newly acquired acceptance, however, I still lacked confidence and would seek approval from others in much of what I did in the classroom. I unconsciously began looking for affection, attention and affirmation, which I found in Doug, my boss.

A coworker of mine eventually told Tom that I was having an affair. My first impulse was to deny it, but I eventually confessed to the truth. He took me to my parents that day, and I stayed with them for some time. Doug ended up resigning as principal.

Tom and I decided to see a counselor. Turns out the counselor's personality assessment classified me as extremely compliant—a category shared with only two percent of the population. It made perfect sense. I had a lifetime of following others in their interests and tabling my own. I really had no idea who I was or what Christine liked and disliked.

Being vocal was so not who I was that I distinctly remember the few times I was vocal. During one of our counseling sessions, I told the pastor about having to get up and leave during our church services to go use the bathroom, despite my prayers to God to take it away.

"That's the MS, not God," I remember him telling me.

"My God is bigger than the MS," I responded resolutely. This I knew.

A new realization soon hit: my students didn't need me like I thought they did. Truth is, any qualified professional could step into my position and my class would be just fine. I was the one who needed them—codependence in action. I thought we both needed each other; and as unhealthy as my thinking was, it was how I saw most relationships. I believed people needed one another so desperately that the life of one simply could not go on without the other. The sad result of this kind of thinking is that I felt externally controlled, and thus helpless.

Then the day that broke my heart came. In a tragic turn of events, my beloved Snickers ran out into the street in front of our home and was hit and instantly killed by a car. I was devastated. I missed his presence in my home. In return, I poured myself into my teaching.

Communication was seriously lacking in my marriage, ultimately ceasing altogether. We found it difficult to agree on what should have been common denominators to our marriage, even my health care options. It wasn't just a matter of arguing for my way; I was now arguing for my health, my life.

In all fairness, relationships are two-sided. And in retrospect, I wonder if it appeared that I magnified the negative and squashed the positive. I'm sure of it. I was insecure and made many mistakes. In my counseling, I learned that no one actually "makes" you feel a certain way. Feelings are a choice, although it certainly doesn't always feel that way.

In hindsight, I realize that I learned to handle conflict by the example set for me growing up - my parents. My dad would get mad and then they wouldn't talk until it somehow blew over. They never seemed to resolve conflicts. I then grew up scared of anger and avoiding conflict at all cost.

Another hindsight lesson I came away with was thinking others knew how I felt, what was wrong and what they should do about it. This caused a lot of problems for a newlywed couple trying to communicate. When Tom asked what was wrong, I thought I explained it but he didn't usually understand or agree. I seemed to always feel guilty for what I said or thought. Then somewhere in my mind I decided that was something I wouldn't bring up again. After a while, there was a lot I wasn't talking about with him. I would just bottle it up.

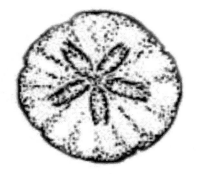

Chapter Nine

Boundaries, Healing & Resolutions

We didn't seem to make a lot of progress in the church counseling, so I went away to Chicago for some individual counseling. It was during this time I finally dealt with my MS diagnosis, which was good for me personally. In my marriage, I had not felt valued as a person.

Counseling taught me to set boundaries with others, something I had never done and something I still struggle with even to this day. The Boundaries® study by Cloud and Townsend was life changing. I did learn to stand up for myself a little better. Tom and I hashed through a lot during this time. After my time in Chicago I felt stronger and more confident.

With the psychological healing from my time at New Life also came spiritual healing. I came to understand a Jesus who was not out to catch or punish me as I had mistakenly thought. Instead, He lived inside me and loved me. What a revelation! My image of God evolved from seeing God "out there" to seeing, feeling and knowing Him to be "in me." I had heard this news before, and I even already knew it, but my mental image of God didn't line up with what I knew—until now.

There was a slight shift in our relationship dynamic, as Tom began to focus less on work and more on our marriage. But it was too late; I was already done. Now I actually had both men fighting for me—my husband and my boss. I felt like I was running nonstop. I'm a pleaser by nature, but this time I was pleasing no one. I couldn't continue like this.

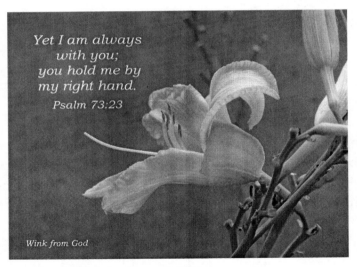

Yet I am always with you; you hold me by my right hand.
Psalm 73:23

Wink from God

Photo by Christine Ganger © 2016

Chapter Ten

Wants & Needs

In February of 2001 I spent three weeks in day counseling at New Life Counseling Center in Illinois. The counselor asked me to make a list of my "wants" and my "needs." This is the list I provided:

My Wants & Needs

1. A family who wants and loves me simply for who I am, not wanting or expecting more
2. Someone who always believes in me
3. Someone who makes me feel safe
4. Someone who makes me feel sexy, exciting and even smart
5. Help and encouragement at school
6. Someone who listens about my past
7. Someone to whom I can tell everything
8. Someone who wants to know everything about me
9. Someone to admire and feel proud of
10. Someone who shares everything with me
11. Incredible memories
12. Someone who encourages me to be me and to grow"

Chapter Eleven

Dear Multiple Sclerosis

I t was now ten years since my diagnosis, and I was finally dealing with my anger and losses from MS. The counselor asked me if I was angry with God.

"No, He's God," I said, which led to my next assignment. Write a letter to my MS. So I did just that; I wrote a letter to my MS. I felt angry as I wrote it, but it wouldn't hit me until I had to read it aloud. I wept.

Letter to Multiple Sclerosis

Dear MS,

 I am very angry with all you took from my life. Yes, I know you could and can still do a lot more damage. I know what you took from me might not look like a big deal to others, but they're not me and they don't live with you day after day reminding them what a klutz they are.

Letter to Multiple Sclerosis continued ...

I hate that I am afraid to have children because I don't want them to be embarrassed by me. I also can't bear the thought of having children and not being able to do all of the things I have dreamed I would do with them, such as playing ball, chasing them and just having fun.

I hate having to go to the bathroom so often. It embarrasses me and makes me angry. I make jokes and laugh so that I don't cry.

Why did you choose me? Some people think their lives begin at the age of 21. I hate that my whole outlook on life changed and became very scary at age 21. You have already taken enough from me —please don't take anymore. I hate all of my daily reminders of you as it is.

To this day, I recommend this letter-writing technique to anybody experiencing loss of any kind, present or past, whether for you, a spouse or loved one, parent or child. It's a safe tool and helps its author deal with and release those feelings. Reading it out loud to someone you trust is essential to gain its full benefit. It can certainly be a challenge to do, but it is well worth it.

Chapter Twelve

Divorce, Beauty & Decisions

The summer of 2001 would prove pivotal for me; just short of our nine-year anniversary, I left my husband. I decided I needed to get away from everyone and think for myself. I hopped in the car, all by my lonesome, and drove out to Montana, the place of my mother's youth and the vacation spot of my childhood. I let both men know before I hit the road what my plans were and that I needed time away. It wasn't fair, or healthy, for me to continue this charade.

Here I was in my parents' car headed to my promised land. It was a long drive from Indiana to my destination in Montana. I took my time. It was a very emotional drive and it took me three days to arrive at my destination.

The area held so many fond memories for me—memories of keeping company with my grandpa, of camping trips in his motorhome, of his teaching me to build fires—oh, how my whole family had loved those times.

I had underlying goals for the trip (i.e., trying to figure out my life and make some major decisions, away from all influences).

The first morning I sat out on my grandma's deck. My grandfather had passed away when I was in high school. I looked out across the lot at his trucking business. I had to smile thinking about rides in the semi-truck with him and great times playing on the equipment with my cousins. I wanted my morning coffee. Even when I was young I could be a bit of a pest, which reminds me of how I developed my love of coffee. Whenever my grandpa would put his coffee cup down, I would grab it and finish it off.

"Christine," he would yell with a smile on his face as he reached for his cup only to find its contents gone missing!

The following day I drove up to Glacier National Park. It was without a doubt the most beautiful place I had ever been. It rained on my drive up; and to my delight I was blessed with the most beautiful rainbow. Once in the park, realizing that I was actually here—against the odds—the tears flowed. I never thought I would see this beauty again, as Tom had no interest in ever making the trip. It was wonderful being there alone. I drove the scenic highways, pulling over every chance I could get, and just gazed upon God's magnificent creation. I was happy to be able to do some hiking while there. My camera instinctively gobbled up every bit of beauty I stumbled upon. I still recollect that time with fondness; it was the most amazing day.

My grandma had been in Ohio for a cousin's wedding during my stay, which laid the groundwork for my time of solitude and afforded the perfect opportunity to get some personal writing and rumination done. In my stillness, I contemplated the direction of my life. I wrote and wrote and wrote. Then I would tear up the pages and burn them. My mind replayed my many mistakes. But ultimately, I was married and no longer loved my husband. And I had found myself in love with another man. I was in the middle of all kinds of lies, but it had to stop. I was a Christian and I knew God loved me, but he could never love the choices I was making. Feeling undeserving, I just wanted to be happy—to feel loved. What would I do?

I was a Christian, but I had become stagnant and had no relationship with Christ or His followers. Up to now, I had been content floating along. But now it was time to make a decision; after my three-week hiatus I called Doug, and he flew out to drive home with me. It was time for a new school year to begin.

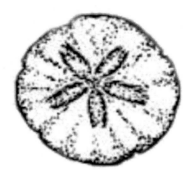

Chapter Thirteen

Excommunication & Shame

I immediately received word from my church that my membership had been revoked. The message arrived via answering machine. The children's pastor listed the charges against me in that humiliating voice message. Apparently because I had chosen to "continue to live in sin," the leaders of the church revoked my membership.

WOW! Want to know what it feels like to get sucker-punched in the gut? That was it. I knew my choices to be with Doug and leave my husband were wrong. I already felt sad and ashamed, and now my dose had doubled. But I wasn't willing to change and go back. I wanted to be with Doug and know love. I chose love. I chose Doug.

Of course now everybody knew the truth. I feared I would never be accepted by any of my friends or people in the church now. We were always looking over our shoulders, and it felt that I wore a big scarlet letter broadcasting my guilt and shame. I thought everyone was talking about how horrible I was and that no one could ever like me or understand my choices.

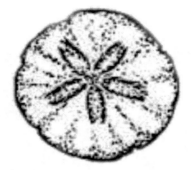

Chapter Fourteen

New Chance at Love

A year later I married Doug—my best friend. We wed in Panama beach, Florida. We opted for an intimate ceremony on the beach, with just the pastor and us. We sat with my parents prior to leaving to tell them about our plans. "I don't think you are asking," my dad said. But ultimately, my mom and dad just wanted me happy.

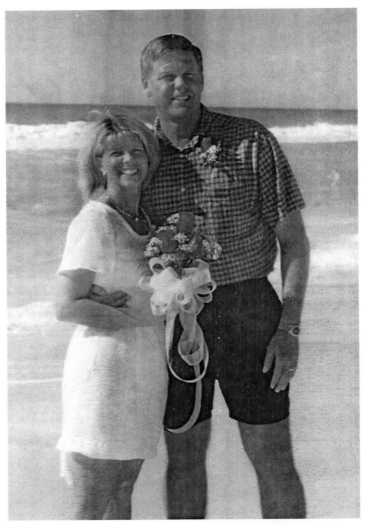

Doug and Christine Ganger
Beach wedding in Panama Beach, Fl.
Photo by Christine Ganger © 2016

Chapter Fifteen

Nowhere To Run

Early on in our marriage, we attended a church that was big enough no one would notice us. Doug was hoping to get back into education and had upcoming interviews in Virginia, Georgia and California. We were hoping to get out of the area and maybe avoid some of the uncomfortable consequences of our choices. Ha! That wasn't God's plan at all. We ended up staying in the same area. I remained teaching at the same school, and Doug ended up getting back into education at an alternative school, a job that he would later discover to be his mission.

I now had a new life, a new home and good friends. And I was once again involved in Bible studies. My heart was full. Doug and I read Rick Warren's Purpose Driven Life together. We prayed a hedge of protection around our marriage, and we helped one another to set boundaries for our new marriage. We worked on affair-proofing our marriage. I was not worried on any sublevel, but we both agreed that it was a smart and necessary plan. I recommended he avoid the temptation to console female coworkers. This might send mixed messages. He could easily advise them to find a female to confide in. He suggested that some of my bantering with men could be misinterpreted as flirting. Interesting, I honestly wouldn't have thought that. And there was the obvious scenario of either of us finding ourselves in a situation in which we are with someone of the opposite sex. Just don't let it happen! So we were ready now, with game plan in place.

Chapter Sixteen

Infections & Tomatoes

As the new school year approached in 2002, I found myself struggling to walk; I simply hadn't the energy to do anything. It was obviously my MS flaring up again. With school about to start, I just wasn't sure how I was going to do it.

We decided to take a short trip to an outlet mall about an hour away and do some school shopping. By the time we got in the vehicle to head home, I felt ill. It was early August, with temperatures in the 90's and high humidity, yet I was freezing. I couldn't stop shivering. My wonderful husband traveled the whole way home with the heater on for me. We eventually made our way to an emergency room, where I was diagnosed with a urinary tract infection. That explained the 103-degree temperature, a first for me. Some additional lab work revealed that I was anemic, which explained why I was so weak and tired.

As I waited out the infection from home, I broke out in a rash and was itching everywhere. My doctor said I was having an allergic reaction to all of the tomatoes I had been eating. I was relieved, but I hated giving up tomatoes.

As a result of my infection and rash, I was about three weeks late starting the school year. Luckily, I had a wonderful sub and she got the year started off great without much assistance. We would go on to become good friends, and I consider her a true gift from God.

Chapter Seventeen

Running from the Past

I t was no easy task living in the same area where my past also lived. I saw friends and family. People had questions. I was remarried, but the divorced Christine is what people saw and talked about. We had damaged our reputations, lost friends and tried to avoid people. It felt awful. But in my pain, I reflected on my own judgmental nature.

There had been a time when I believed that anyone who had done the things I had done couldn't possibly get to Heaven. I wouldn't have dreamed that I would even know or befriend anybody who could do what I ended up doing. And now, here I was wanting and expecting others to forgive and accept me. Stephen R. Covey once wrote, "We see the world, not as it is, but as we are—or, as we are conditioned to see it." That was me. Because I would have looked at divorced, unfaithful Christine with contempt, it was only natural that others were looking at Christine with the same judgment, right? But to my delight and gratefulness, I discovered that not everyone thought that way. Especially my new church family. They genuinely do not treat anyone's past as an issue—they just want everyone to know Jesus.

Still, Doug and I made some poor choices that came with consequences. I don't want to dwell on this but I need to say these consequences were many, some of which might have lifelong repercussions. We accept the responsibility of our choices and have no one else to blame. I think it was at this point in my life I realized that we make our own choices. And with our choices, we either reap the benefits or pay the consequences. But we must own that byproduct of choice.

Chapter Eighteen

Forgiveness

I ended up needing to apologize and ask forgiveness of a lot of people. This is a letter I sent to some very close friends. It was difficult to send.

I didn't get much feedback from them, but that was all right. I needed to do the right thing by admitting my wrong and being open with them. I now knew God still loved and forgave me. And that is what He wants from me: to love and forgive others.

We moved on with our lives, eventually moving to the lake and joining a small group. We were now mending relationships with family and making new friends.

Nov. 11, 2002

Dear friends,

I know it has been a long time since I have spoken with any of you. My life has changed a lot in this past year and a half.

As all of you know, Tom and I are divorced and I have remarried. All of you have been my true friends for a long time. I am sorry that you had to hear this from someone other than me.

I have gone through some intense counseling and have changed a lot. I had become a person that I didn't like at all. I should have gone to you but I was ashamed and I was afraid no one could understand. I am very sorry for that.

My parents were very disappointed and devastated by the choices I made. My relationship with them has finally recovered. They have seen that I am very happy and am back to being "me."

I do blame my MS for changing me some but there were also many other variables and bad choices. I can say that I am very happy now, and I know you would all agree that my husband is wonderful.

I am hoping that we can reconcile our friendships but also understand if you are unable to do so.

Tom and I ended our relationship on as good of terms as possible. I am very thankful that Doug and I have a wonderful, open relationship. I am also thankful that God never gives up or ever stops loving us. What an incredible God He is!

Love, Christine

Chapter Nineteen

Disney World & A Lake Party

In 2005 I finished my master's degree with help and encouragement from my husband. I don't enjoy taking classes and writing papers. Doug did enjoy those things, however; and he kindly helped me, so it all worked out. In January of 2006 I reached a high point of my teaching. I saw that a local television station had a reading contest for students and the "most creative teacher" would win a trip to Disney World.

"I want to go to Disney World!" I told Doug. So my adorable husband made me a prop for my classroom and I got busy. I made a monthly reading incentive chart that would enable my students to read and track their progress. There would be prizes for individual students who read the most minutes and for classrooms that read the most. And the Mickey Mouse prize would be awarded to the teacher who was most creative in inspiring his or her students to read.

I continued my morning exercise routine. It has always been important for me and essential for living with MS, keeping my muscles strong and maintaining my mobility. The exercises were not really difficult, but they were enough to keep me active.

Twelve months later, Doug and I were in Orlando, Florida, spending New Year's Eve 2007 at Disney World! I had won the contest. The day I found out, I had the class taking a spelling test and in walked a man, followed by a television cameraman, who presented me with a big check. When he announced that I had won the trip to Disney, my students misunderstood and thought the whole class was going! Their misguided excitement was bittersweet, as I told them that their prize would be a big party at my house on the lake. It wasn't Disney World, but a kid can have a lot of fun on a lake! Everybody was happy.

The Disney trip was wonderful—what a way to usher in the new year! Even with my morning rider exercises still a regular part of my daily routine, the walking required at a Disney theme park is fierce and it got the better of me, regardless. We eventually rented a park wheelchair—sitting my pride aside for the day—and enjoyed our time without any risk of my getting exhausted and thus frustrated. It was a big help, indeed!

Chapter Twenty

A Pacemaker for the What?

The next milestone for us as a couple was being asked to be marriage counselors by and for our church. We probably seemed an unlikely choice, given our history, but our experiences had equipped us well for this ministry, and our hearts were ready. Perhaps we might help others avoid making the same mistakes we had.

Doug and I started traveling some on school breaks, but my bladder issues were getting worse. I was visiting the bathroom between eight and 15 times per night, and sleep was something I could only dream about. When I finally saw a urologist, he told me that my case was extreme—not something you want to hear from a doctor! He suggested I try a new procedure that he felt might be a good fit for me.

After a challenging weekend getaway in February 2008, I decided on no more humiliation and struggle with bladder issues. I gave my urologist consent to try the new procedure. At this point I would try anything.

He put in an Interstim (a pacemaker for the bladder), and it did help with the urgency and frequency. I had told the doctor I wanted to be able to walk on the beach with my husband, which had not been possible because by the time we would get to the beach, I already needed to find a bathroom.

That same summer, my MS started flaring up again, so I asked my neurologist if I could go on steroids. They had worked well for me in the past. My doctor said no, but suggested I try the new drug.

I started monthly Tysabri infusions in September 2008. And with the exception that my veins were non-cooperative, my body responded well. To fix the vein problem, a port was inserted, and from then on the process was little more than a little poke each month.

One of the sweet blessings that came out of my monthly infusions was my girlfriend time with Ann, an old teacher friend of mine. Since her retirement from teaching, we had found it difficult to get together. Since my infusion therapy required that I commit at least two hours to being there on the premises, I asked Ann if she would keep me company during this time and she was glad to agree.

After a half day of work, I would check in for treatment. Ann and I would have lunch and then just sit and talk as the IV drained. She is always a wonderful listener and careful not to judge, two incredibly valuable attributes I welcomed from a friend. My time with Ann was truly a gift.

By the end of the year, I was seeing the results of the Interstim, along with the infusions. I could actually walk the beach with Doug now.

Chapter Twenty-One

Progress Report

An email I sent to friends and family July 2, 2009:

To those of you who have been thinking of me and praying for me starting the new MS treatment, I want to share my latest progress.

I can jog in place. I know it sounds like no big deal to most of you, but it's OK. For me, the final summit would be to someday be able to run – it's been 20 years (although I can't say I enjoyed it when I could).

As of this week, I also now walk backward. That allows me to have "eyes in the back of my head" when teaching.

I just wanted to say thanks for your prayers. Praise God, He answers prayer!

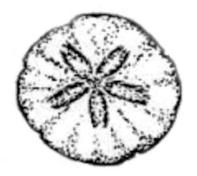

Chapter Twenty-Two

Doctor's Orders

Two years later I went to see my neurologist for my yearly check-up. I expected him to say, "Everything is going well. Continue with the infusions." Instead, he urged me to take a holiday from the meds for a while. I wasn't ready to heed his advice just yet, however. My research could not find any supporting corroboration for going off the medicine. I had never disagreed with a doctor before, being the compliant woman that I was, but I felt this was too important not to. And it felt good, like I was a "big girl" and taking care of myself. It just so happens my cousin had been part of the original testing of the drug and had great success with it. She later had to go off of it for a short time, and when she went back on it her body refused it. I couldn't take that chance.

Chapter Twenty-Three

Mother's Day

I had always struggled with Mother's Day, after making my decision not to have children. I hated the commercials and going to church on that day. I bought into the lie that if you're not a mom, you can't be a wonderful woman. I know I would have been a good mom. In fact, I've played the role at work every day as a teacher. I felt bad for my mom because I wanted to have no part of the celebrations of Mother's Day. It was so unfair to her.

As Mother's Day approached, and as I worked myself into my little funk, Doug caught me off guard. I still didn't like conflict and would avoid it if possible, but Doug was patient and persistent. He didn't mind that we might disagree at times, but he urged me to talk about what bothered me so we could move forward.

"What is it you want or need from me to help you through this time?" I didn't know. I thought about it.

"If I have to tell you, doesn't that kind of discount it?" I thought to myself. If I don't know how can I expect him to know?

After putting some serious thought behind his question, I knew the answer.

"I want you to tell me I would be a great mom and I am like a mom to my students every day."

"That is exactly what I think," Doug said, "and I thought I told you that often."

I wasn't sure, but I knew at Mother's Day that is what I wanted to hear. And so my wonderful husband bought me a beautiful Mother's Day card and wrote those very sentiments inside it, and he has continued that small but precious ritual to me every Mother's Day since.

That little conversation was a life changer for me. I am so grateful he asked the question and was then willing to listen. But the life lesson it taught me was this: How can I expect others to know what I need if I don't even know? Or if I don't tell them?

Chapter Twenty-Four

Grandchildren

While I had made the decision early on to not have children of my own, I still managed to end up being a mom—a stepmom to my husband, Doug's, two adult children.

August 10, 2009, was one of the hardest days of my life. Our daughter-in-law was in labor for 36 hours—OK, so it wasn't an easy time for her either! As this new life inched its way to this side of humanity, the impact of my early decision hit with great magnitude. This would be the closest I would ever come to being a part of bringing new life into this world, and the reality of the situation struck me with a hard blow. I wept uncontrollably all day, questioning whether I had made the right choice, wondering how things could have been. My heart bled years of bottled-up emotions and longings that day. The pain was nearly unbearable.

But joy came in the morning—at 12:30 a.m. to be exact. Our grandson will never know the healing he brought into my life. As a woman, I always felt a void because of not being a mom or having children. But being a grandmother to this new little life was an experience of equal magnitude and wonder.

Our second precious grandson was born in February 2011—a double blessing of joy. Being a grandparent is everything and more.

Chapter Twenty-Five

Hard Decisions

In the summer of 2011, my neurologist wanted to run a test on me for a virus that had the potential to do much damage and even proving fatal to some. I had been receiving monthly infusions for five years now, and my MS seemed to be at bay.

I tested positive for the possibility of a previous JC virus exposure, which prompted my doctor to urge me to go off of the infusions (continuing them could subject me to possible brain disease).

This was a big decision for me. It would be the first time I'd tackle such a monumental decision without the input from others. Normally I would have welcomed the advice of others, but I realized that no one else had any input. Surprisingly, I found myself upset with Doug for chiming in on the topic. I knew that the percentage of those who had become fatally ill from the drug was small, and I knew I had achieved a quality of life with it that I hadn't had prior to the infusions.

As I became a stronger person and gained more confidence in myself, I was able to make what I felt was the best decision for me. With Doug's support, I told my doctor I would not go off of the infusions. Some comfort I found as I made my decision:

"Your eyes saw my unformed body; all the days ordained for me were written in your book before one of them came to be." ~Psalm 139:16 NIV

I realized my days were numbered before I was born, and this decision wasn't going to add or take away from it. So continue, I did.

Chapter Twenty-Six

Shingles

Infusions continued and all was well, until the Monday before Thanksgiving of 2011 when something strange happened. I was standing in the hallway talking with some coworkers after work, when suddenly I felt something in my hip and fell straight to the ground.

That was the first incident of what would be the start of a bad downhill cycle. It was now common for me to get these pains and just fall. I made an appointment with my neurologist to find out what was going on. The day before my appointment as I put my socks on, I noticed a rash on my right calf. I had come down with shingles!

Because of the numbness attributed to MS and not having much feeling in my legs, I didn't notice any irritation from the Shingles. Therefore I didn't experience the pain that accompanies shingles. On the other hand, without the MS, we might have caught the Shingles earlier and lessoned the damage that was to follow.

Christine Ganger

An Email to a Friend Dec 02, 2011:

Hey Friends, Just thought I would give you a little "'heads up" on what is happening. Well, really I don't know but...it all started Tuesday at the end of the school day. My hip started giving out and I was falling. Since then, it has become weaker and more painful - I really can't walk at all. I went in yesterday for a CAT scan hoping to rule out the BAD side effect of my medicine. I haven't received a call from the doctor yet with the results. Just thought I would let you know what is happening. I have no fear right now only peace but I welcome your prayers.
Thanks for your concern and support!

Subject: RE: FYI
Praise GOD! The doctor just called and it is not the MS or PML. Now tears of JOY. Thanks!

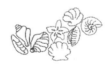

Chapter Twenty-Seven

A Second Spinal Tap

Earlier that fall, there was a gal doing her student teaching just down the hall from me. We became good friends. She was just finishing up her student teaching and moved right in to substitute teach for my class. I was out a lot the next couple of months. The Shingles rash cleared up, but I became weaker and struggled to walk at all.

Because of my Interstim, an MRI was not an option, so they wanted to do a spinal tap—the second one in my lifetime. It would give a more accurate synopsis than the CAT scan I'd had. I remember telling Doug that I would never get a spinal tap again, not after the horrible repercussions I suffered from my first one years earlier. But they needed to rule out the JC virus; my doctor thought that was probably what I had.

I had the spinal tap on December 23, 2011. I wholeheartedly leaned on the 23rd Psalm:

"Yea, though I walk through the valley of the shadow of death, I will fear no evil: for thou art with me; thy rod and thy staff they comfort me."
~Psalm 23:4 KJV

Praise God they have made tremendous improvement sense that ill-fated spinal tap I'd received years earlier. Finally, on December 27, I got the test back; it was negative.

Chapter Twenty-Eight

Isolation

The Shingles had done some lasting damage, especially to my hips. I participated in Physical therapy twice a week. I went in the morning and then would go work for the rest of the day. It was so hard. I'm not sure it was a good idea to go to work afterward.

I had gotten my grandma's electric scooter to use at work. Everything was worse—I was falling more often and my right foot dragged all the time. Discouraged and self-conscious, I wouldn't go anywhere without Doug. My strength and stamina were so weak that everything was difficult. With my right foot dragging, I would trip over rugs or catch my foot on the floor and fall.

I went through a couple rounds of physical therapy. I took on the habit of grazing—hugging walls and/or people as a means of defense from falling. The problem with grazing is that walls might stay put but the other things I grabbed onto didn't necessarily oblige. So every now and then, down I went!

I wouldn't go to a store by myself. I would park in a handicap spot but I didn't even have the strength to make it from the car into the store, so there was no sense in trying. When we did shop together, I always held Doug's arm, or we would get a wheelchair. I was embarrassed someone might see me in the wheelchair, but it helped us accomplish what we needed. Of course, being seen in a wheelchair was still far better than being seen falling flat on the ground.

I was usually good just staying home. Trying to appear strong was exhausting. I really wanted to believe I could hide how weak and tired I was, but I couldn't. Besides battling fatigue, I battled humiliation. I wanted to be around people, but that took effort and I really wasn't even able to engage with others because I was so distracted.

I realized through all of this that my priorities no longer resembled those of any of my friends. While they concerned themselves with matters of what to wear, shopping, holiday meals, getting yard work or housework done, and such, I just wanted to have the strength to be with others. My health was my only concern.

Daily tasks turned into strategic productions for me. I pre-planned the most efficient but least resistant routes before I embarked on any adventure. I ended up missing a lot of work during this time and being home by myself. And another realization I had was how everyone's lives were going on without me. I felt insignificant; but at the same time, I realized how much I needed people—interacting, socializing, and making friends.

We discussed at length my going on disability, but I would work hard to not let that happen.

The physical therapy helped—especially the stationary bike, which they insisted would help strengthen my hips. I even later bought a stationary bike to use at home. Now my workouts would alternate between the rider and the bike.

Through the spring and summer I had regained some of my strength and balance. When school started in the fall I no longer used a cane regularly and happily returned the scooter to my grandma. I didn't walk great, but I was determined to push forward.

Chapter Twenty-Nine

Letter to Paul Young

April 25, 2012, The Shack author Paul Young, came and spoke to our church. This is an email I wrote to him after the service. I had an "Aha" of understanding God's love in a way I never had before. God will always say, "I still love you!"

This is the email I sent to Paul Young after the service:

> I have MS and never had children of my own but my husband has two. I know why God gave me grandchildren – to help me understand how encompassing HIS love is.

Continued ...

After your message I can better relate to this and that He still loves me and just wants to be with me – or me be with Him. I just relate it to how no matter what my grandson does – I still love him, I want to just be with him. This has truly been a gift.

I woke up thinking God was so excited I was awake so he could show me His beautiful painting in the sky. I can now understand that God would love for me just to talk with him and not waste time on my computer.

Chapter Thirty

New Job Assignment

In May 2012, I was ready to get out of the classroom and do something different. A new interventionist position opened at our school. It sounded perfect. I would work in small groups with kids struggling to read. I had been watching and had even applied for some other positions but nothing worked out. When our principal asked if anyone was interested, of course I jumped on it. I even went one step further, going in and telling her why I thought I should get it. I now had my master's in special education and had been a reading coach in the past.

I got the job, and I am so thankful for it. I believe God wrote this job description just for me. With the new job came a different kind of commitment for support from me to the other teachers that had never been necessary. I was now interacting with teachers on behalf of their students, listening to their specific concerns about each child and then working with each child to meet the challenges and concerns as agreed. It also felt good to just walk in a classroom and assist when needed. I know as a classroom teacher how much I would have appreciated someone coming in and just seeing what was needed without judging me. I loved my new role!

Chapter Thirty-One

Adventure

My adventurer status from my youthful days might have appeared lost, but I knew I still had it in me. Doug was happy letting me plan vacations for the two of us; I've always loved to travel. And I've always wanted to go to see the rain forest, so I planned a spring break adventure to Costa Rica for us and two other couples. None of us had been before. I was so excited. I like having a "carrot" out there to look forward to, so I reserved a home that September. I let everyone know I intended to experience some adventure on this trip.

Costa Rica was beautiful. Most of the time we just enjoyed being around the pool. The adventures were very nice but we saved the big one for last. I had made some calls prior to arriving and did some research on zip lining. I was determined to do it but there had to be an option that didn't require a lot of walking. So we purchased a package called "Extreme Adventure," which included an afternoon riverboat sightseeing adventure, an evening sunset cruise and a day of horseback riding to the top of a mountain with a zip line ride back down. I was so excited!

We got up early, rode to a nice place for breakfast and then off to the stables. We mounted our horses and road 45 minutes up a mountain. They gave us the how-to crash course as we strapped ourselves into our gear. We would have 10 different zip line runs before we reached the end. I wasn't one of the first ones to go, but I was very eager. When strapping up, I felt the guide was treating me a bit gingerly. I don't walk well and I am weak, but still I don't like to be treated as though I'm frail.

The first ride was awesome! Doug went in front of me in case I needed his help on the landings. As I was getting hooked up for the second run I told the guide I wanted to go upside down. He looked a bit surprised and then smiled. He agreed. As I neared the platform I could see Doug. He had a big grin on his face. He shook his head and I heard him say, "That's my girl!" The whole experience was just great!

Parasailing is the next adventure on my "Bucket List."

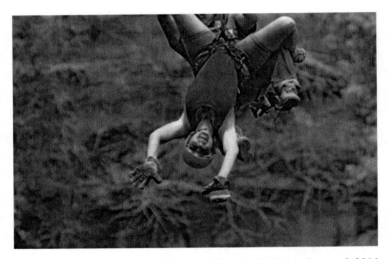

Photo by Christine Ganger © 2016

Chapter Thirty-Two

My Gift

I continued on the Infusions for another year when my liver count went up. I was now seeing a new neurologist and he didn't give me the option to continue. Soon I needed my cane on a more regular basis.

Whenever Doug and I were together, we would walk arm in arm. I felt very secure when I was with him. This helped me with my balance and kept me from tiring out so quickly.

Doug is a strong man, which comes in handy when I get tired. But the beauty of Doug stretched far beyond his mere strength. He had this way of knowing me – of anticipating my moves – that gave me great comfort. With my bladder issues still front and center, I had to always know where a bathroom was at any given time. And when I felt the need to get to the bathroom, there was no "later," it was always "right now." And there's this phenomenon that would happen when I tried to split my focus between my bladder and my legs. It was like a switch in my brain that only allowed one of those functions to be in the "on" position at any given time. If I focused heavily on getting to a bathroom, which was no inconsequential feat, I would experience weakness in my legs and my gate suffered. What average person could understand such a crazy thing? Doug understands it perfectly, and never requires any explanation from me. He is such a gift.

Facebook Post: January 12, 2013

Just a little "wake up call" I would like to share with everyone. SLOW DOWN and realize your blessings. I have felt like I've been doing this with trying to capture some of God's beautiful creation in pictures but.

This morning we were babysitting our grandsons (a little side note for those who do not know me I have MS and have had no children of my own. So, just having these little boys who call me grandma is a HUGE blessing alone!)

Because of my MS, I stagger some when I walk. Today we were playing Hide & Seek and my grandson, who is only 3 said, "Are you okay? Come on. You can hold my hand." At the time I thought it was cute and went on playing the game with them.

Now I think about it and get very emotional. How sweet of a little boy to think of helping me by holding my hand and walking with me! It easy to just keep moving to the "next thing" or worrying about whatever is on our plate and miss those beautiful blessing!

I know this is a bit lengthy but... take some time today and acknowledge all your blessings!! God is GOOD all the time!

Chapter Thirty-Three

Hope Resurfaces

In February 2014 my doctor informed me that my MS was now Secondary Progressive. This usually means a more steadily progressive phase of the disease characterized by greater nerve damage or loss. The only treatment option they gave me was a three-day steroid blast. I felt good about that option, since it had worked well for me in the past.

This time was different, however. The treatment made me sick, and my doctor's reaction was little more than, "sorry, there is nothing more we can do at this time."

I still tried to do my rider each morning, but it became harder and I was very weak before I even headed out to work each day.

I became depressed and began to lose hope, and hope had been a huge catalyst for me. The last time I had felt any semblance of hopelessness had been years earlier in my first marriage. That was the darkest, ugliest place I had ever been.

And Yet God would again show Himself to be good and faithful. I started a new business adventure with a nice camera Doug had blessed me with the previous year; I called it Wink from God. I was able to take my studies from the Bible and combine them with beautiful photographs, turning them into framed art and greeting cards. Friends and family bought my scripture art from me. I even built a website for my art.

From my Wink from God Facebook page

> This is a new adventure for us. Just a couple months ago my sister was going through a difficult time and it was her birthday. I wanted to get her a meaningful gift, not just a sweater. I couldn't find anything, so I prayed and asked God to help me find something "meaningful." Just a few days later I woke up with this idea I know was from God and have gone a bit crazy with it.
>
> God has opened my eyes to see His creation like I never have before! Through this I have really dove into the Bible and found incredible things I never knew were there.
>
> I've always thought that my spiritual gift was encouragement. I am so excited to spread encouragement and hope to you and others through God's creation and His word. May God Bless you, and I hope you enjoy!

Though my business never actually took off, it kept me busy and in a better headspace. I made several art donations to help local charities, which in turn auctioned off my pieces. I was hopeful the photos and meaningful verses would encourage others, help the charities and possibly be an investment in eternity.

"The LORD will fight for you; you need only to be still." ~Exodus 14:14 NIV

This Bible verse is one of the nuggets that I wish I'd stumbled upon much earlier in life. It might have made some difference. If I had trusted God to fight for me instead of insisting on fighting for myself, might the results have been different?

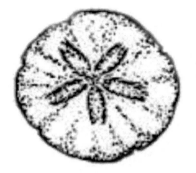

Chapter Thirty-Four

Weight Gain

My depression put added pounds on me; I was eating without abandon. I developed a wicked sweet tooth and craved cream-filled Long John doughnuts paired with a type of flavored coffee from Seven Eleven—we affectionately called them "Co-Nuts" for short. Doug, with his sweet, accommodating self, frequently called me on his way home to see if I needed a "Co-Nut" fix. Such a sweet, little enabler! The sweets led to salt cravings, and a vicious cycle was born. I knew I was gaining weight, but I would stay in denial as long as I avoided the scales.

I became weaker; it all took so much effort. I would come home from work and retire on the couch in my comfy pajamas with laptop, phone, and Bible in hand. Doug was now fixing most of our meals and doing all the work around the house. He continued to love me and tell me I was beautiful, but I knew how I looked in the mirror and I was no longer the girl he had married. Still, he had a way of making me feel loved and beautiful. The way he looked at me—his gaze told a love story that I could not deny. He never stopped wanting to touch me, hold my hand and be near me.

But as wonderful as Doug was to me, it had been a long time since I felt pretty. I tried hard to look my best with cute clothes and makeup but was sure that once I stood and people saw me walk, I wasn't pretty at all.

Chapter Thirty-Five

I Get By
with a Little Help from
My Friends

I love fishing in the spring. We are blessed to live on a lake. It's one of the luxuries that Doug and I decided early in our marriage that we wanted to work hard to have and share together. This spring was the first ever in which fishing was no longer fun for me. The 30-yard walk to the water was met with falls—even with the help of my walker. I felt so sad and discouraged.

Summer came and I developed yet another odd symptom. I would get a stomachache every time I consumed fruit or coffee. I didn't bother the doctor about it; I was sure it would blow over. But instead of blowing over, it forced me to give up both fruit and coffee, two of my favorite things, for the summer. The timing was horrible, as it was the summer that my parents' bucket list wish of taking an Alaskan cruise would come to fruition, and Doug and I would join them. Who goes on a cruise and can't eat all the free yummy foods?

I returned to school in August 2014 and struggled to do much of my job. I made the effort each day, going to work and climbing the stairs three times per day. My friends at work were wonderful, and they were always willing to help me—if only I would ask. When you don't want to be seen as helpless, you tend not to ask for help. That was my reality.

What most people didn't know was how horrible the mornings were for me. Heat is a major issue with MS. If I showered and dried my hair in the morning, I was left weak and unable to walk. My doctors, however, urged me to work out in the mornings since that is the time I would be fresh. I saw the merit in their argument and would do my best to make it happen.

I would fall many times before even getting in the car for work. I called them "soft falls." I Thank God I could usually catch myself with my hands out in front of me. I don't know how I got through all of the falls with no big problems. I would fall in the bathroom because my hips were so weak. Going from standing to sitting and then back up was very difficult. I often would catch myself with my head against the wall. Sometimes just one knee would give out, and down I would go. And going down was the easy part; the getting up was a bear. Once I recovered from a fall and was standing again, I would be worn out and in need of rest.

Curbs were especially tough. I would overthink the height and not be able to lift my foot high enough or not straighten my leg to bring the other one up. And winter had its own set of problems. Canes slide on ice! I fell on the ice before school once, and there was no way that my body was going to let me get up on my own. Fortunately one of my co-teachers pulled up and helped me up and into the building. Tenacity looks like stubbornness when you don't want to give up, but it looks like pride when you let that kind of incident humiliate you.

By the time I got to school, I felt as if I had already put in a day's work; I was exhausted. But God had given me this job that I love and was extremely thankful for, and I knew He would give me the strength to do that job. I needed to smile and be happy! I would do my job while loving and encouraging others!"

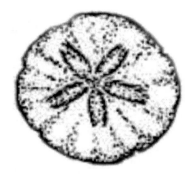

Chapter Thirty-Six

Positivity As Catalyst

The previous school year I had started sending a school-wide email to staff. The purpose of the email was to encourage others. Let's face it; it was certainly easy to get discouraged and be negative at work. I was hoping this might help encourage everyone—starting with me. I called it Positive Connection.

Below is an email I sent to staff:

> Good morning! It's another Thursday to be thankful and share good news.
>
> Each week it is great hearing so many good things from so many. Please continue to share the "good" in your life.
>
> I am very thankful to be starting my 20th year of teaching. This is with much thanks to our wonderful staff. I realize I haven't pulled my weight the past couple of years with my weakness increasing. Starting tomorrow, I will keep a scooter here at school to help me do my job better and hopefully leave me with enough energy for my evenings at home …

Cont...

This is a hard step for me! It feels like I am giving up, but I also realize it is pride that has kept me from taking this step sooner. I hope now I can perform all my duties better with few limitations.

THANKS for bearing with me up until this point. As you know with my MS diagnosis before my student teaching, I never thought I would ever teach! God still performs miracles – Keep your eyes wide open. ☺

This email was very hard to send; it made me cry. I really think that God needed me to deal with my pride issue before I could move forward.

A coworker once asked me how I "keep the faith."

"It's not an option," I said. "That is what keeps me moving."

Shortly afterward at church our pastor talked about how important worship is. Even when you don't feel like it, you need to sing and worship God in order to move closer to Him. That same evening I pondered his words, wondering how my coworker and some other friends are in what seems to be hopeless places. I tried to think of how or why they would worship God in a time like that, especially when there had been no relationship with him prior to their circumstances.

As I slept I had a very real dream in which I had been talking to God and asked Him how people in bad places should or would worship. God replied in a very strong but simple voice, "Faith, Hope and Love." I got it and understood. I am still in awe of this. Only in Him can we have faith, hope and unconditional love.

"A positive attitude causes a chain reaction of positive thoughts, events and outcomes. It is a catalyst and it sparks extraordinary results."
~Wade Boggs

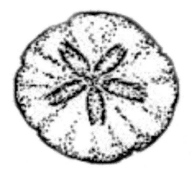

Chapter Thirty-Seven

Hope Springs from the Sunshine State

My mom took a trip back to Montana in 2014 for my aunt's funeral and ended up staying to care for my grandma. Little did I know that this beautiful state would once again be the catalyst for change in my life.

While there, mom ran into a lady she had met before. On her previous visit, the woman had been wheelchair-bound and very ill; this trip, she was not. She was fine, in fact.

The woman told mom about a man in Florida she had visited who made her better. She also shared the testimonies of others who had experienced great health results from this guy. One of those testimonies was that of the woman's sister—who just so happened to have MS!

I got the contact info from my mom and called this Godsend myself for more information.

"His treatment might seem very 'hokey,' but do whatever he says," she said. Then she went on to explain how she had erred at the beginning by not following his precise instruction and ended up wasting a lot of time

By the way, I'm in Michigan. My mom was in Montana and this miracle man is in Florida. Who else but God could bring us together like that?

So what was all of this going to cost, and should I give this guy a chance? Surely it would cost upward of $10,000. And if so, we couldn't do it. My parents were excited about the possibility and the hope it brought. They were even willing to pitch in for the cause, if it came to that. I love them for it, but I could never ask them to make that kind of financial sacrifice.

I discovered the three-day visit would be $2,000, and it just happened that that was exactly what I had in my HSA account (money to be used for medical purposes). So I had them put me on his call list; and to my amazement, that Friday evening the doctor, Jack, called me.

"I love MS," he told me. Seriously, I have never heard those words used together!

"There's a three-month waiting list; but because I love MS, I'll put you on the cancellation wait-list," he told me. That would mean I was fourth on the list. I was so excited. Why not? I had nothing to lose, and my MS doctor said that there was nothing more he could do for me at this time. Here was my ticket to explore—to look for something more. In one of our conversations, Jack tried to explain using frequencies in treatment to me, but I didn't understand how that could work in healing the body.

"How did you come up with this?" I asked him.

"It had to be the Holy Spirit," he answered. That was the moment I knew I wanted him on my team.

I must have walked on air as I waited to make the trip to see him. Additionally, spending January in Florida sounded pretty good as we headed into our winter season. Doug and I were even willing to make whatever adjustments to our diet that were necessary; his plan was to adapt for himself whatever diet, no matter how rigorous, the doctor would require of me. Such a good sport.

The countdown was on. I even set a countdown app on my phone. Then in early October I came home to a message on my phone from the clinic.

"We have an opening October 13, can you come?"

Suddenly my countdown shrank from 92 days to 10! Most of our friends and family were extremely supportive, with prayers coming from practically everyone we knew. What a complete blessing from God this was. And while some people voiced their suspicions and concerns about the treatment, we chose to override them. Yes, we did not let their fear take root in us. It all actually felt like a surprise vacation dropped right into our laps!

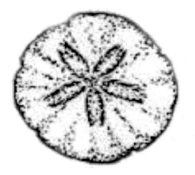

Chapter Thirty-Eight

Priorities in Saint Augustine

We left on a Friday and arrived in St. Augustine late Saturday night. The weather forecast was perfect for the week. Having heard of the beauty in our nation's oldest city, we decided to take our time and look around before checking in to the office Monday morning, especially given the fact that we had no idea how I would feel during or after the treatments. I had to start the detoxing procedures 36 hours before I was to begin the treatment—that meant no caffeine, sugar or dairy.

Our hotel wasn't far from the beach, so our plan was to take a few walks during our stay. Robyn, one of my coaches from high school, lived in the area and volunteered to show us around. We met up and had a great day. She was the one who inspired me to put my journey to paper. She encouraged me to do this because she felt God was in the midst of writing a great story to share.

When Monday morning finally rolled around, we found our way to the office. It was far from fancy, but that was fine with me. We were the only ones there with Dr. Jack and his two assistants. A patient was finishing up when we came, and then the following appointment was there when we left—a pattern that repeated with each of our visits. It was a pretty orderly system. Not like the typical doctor's office filled with helpless, frustrated, double-booked patients waiting well beyond their scheduled time slot to see the doctor.

Upon first meeting Jack, we were very comfortable. He sat at his desk across from me, and Doug sat next to me.

"Multiple Sclerosis just means many viruses," Jack told us.

"We need to find the viruses and get them out of your body."

"Then let's get busy," I blurted out.

I had filled out paperwork before we arrived, listing all past procedures and medications. He also had me list my top three priorities. While most people would think my first priority would have been mobility, it was not; my No. 1 priority was my bladder. I no longer had complete control over it and had to wear adult pull-ups. This admission was probably the most humbling of my lifetime. If you can't relate to this issue, then I would encourage you to thank God; and in the same breath, pray that you never will. My second and third priorities were balance and mobility.

I spent the first two hours with my foot on Jack's knee. Relax; it's not what it seems! He used this yellow wand to tap on my toes as a computer simultaneously ran diagnostics on me, producing a list of the various viruses, toxins and metals it found in my body. I watched Jack attack each of the intruders with frequencies that I couldn't actually feel, but I saw the numbers falling and I trusted the computer readouts.

I spent the next two hours with straps around my ankles and wrist and a goofy contraption on my head. I was expected to enter specific frequencies written out for me into a machine and for a specific amount of time.

In his wisdom, Jack was able to diagnose a thyroid problem in me as soon as he saw me.

" How do you know that?" I asked him. "You just now met me." Turns out my dry skin gave me away. He suggested I take iodine, and then later would add Iodine co-factors to my order. My skin is much softer as a result.

And remember all the stomach pain I had been getting every time I ate fruit? He said it was because I was full of yeast. Apparently when the yeast and sugar mix, they make a nice little alcohol cocktail. Our bellies are like mini breweries churning out alcohol. I was given two grapefruit seed extract tablets: one to chew and one to swallow. And lo and behold, it worked!

I now know it is called candida. My family doctor said that there's no test for candida in western medicine. I was happy to be able to pass on my newfound knowledge to a couple of friends who had been having the same symptoms, and they, too, found relief once I shared the remedy.

Doug and I had lunch afterward and went back to the hotel. Feeling the need to rest, I napped for a couple of hours. I was delighted to wake up feeling well, so we spent the evening going for dinner and a walk to the beach.

I didn't sleep well that night, but I didn't expect I would. Jack warned me of possible detox symptoms. I was up several times throughout the night for my regular bathroom visits, plus my body ached.

I left Jack's office with three spray bottles in hand: one for inflammation, one for chemicals and the third for drainage. The detox could look different from person to person; some have stomach issues, some have gas or diarrhea. I was to apply the drainage spray to whatever part of my body felt discomfort, along with three squirts under the tongue. I was instructed to use the chemical spray at least day and night, with three squirts under the tongue and then on various points of my head.

I used the sprays a lot that night. I think it helped some, but I couldn't be sure. The next day was about the same as the first.

My Facebook post at the end of my first day with Dr. Jack:

October 13, 2014 ·
    I had a four-hour treatment today. Still feeling encouraged but very tired. Need to rest up. It will be the same thing the next couple days. Nothing new to share yet.
    Thank you for the prayers and please keep them coming— feeling drained.

Facebook Post: October 15, 2014

"I was feeling discouraged this morning before my appointment but was encouraged by my prayer partners. Now my treatments are finished and I/we are very encouraged. I believe the doctor finished finding everything there was to find and treated them. I will continue the virus blast over the next couple days and weeks. My walking seems to have already improved some and so has my twitching. The doctor has done his part, now I will do mine by following the doctor's protocol. Praising God because I know He will continue to do His part. PRAISING GOD!!"

This is my treatment each day after meeting with the doctor and him doing his thing. I am punching in frequencies to kill viruses in my body. Yes, I know it looks strange, but I believe I'm getting better.

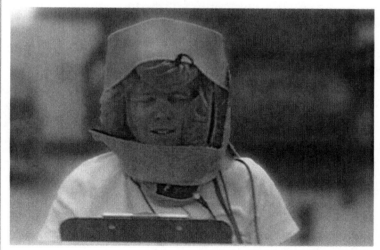

Photo by Christine Ganger © 2016

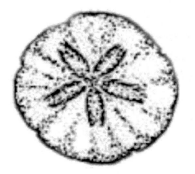

Chapter Thirty-Nine

Home & Liquid Gold

J ack instructed me as to which supplements I must take. I was to continue with the grapefruit seed extract as needed, along with a probiotic. I was also instructed to take Primrose and Black Currant oil. This was to help repair the myelin sheath that Multiple Sclerosis is known to destroy.

After my three days of treatment with Dr. Jack, we got up early on day No. 4 and went down to the beach to watch the sunrise. It was beautiful. We spent the rest of the day in St. Augustine. We went to the lighthouse. I did more walking that day then I had done in a long time, although I didn't climb the 400+ steps to the top of the lighthouse. Doug did, however, and paid dearly for it the next day.

We made it home tired but hopeful. Doug was now hurting from the lighthouse walk followed by the long ride home. I suggested he try the inflammation spray Jack gave me. Surely, it couldn't hurt. So he tried it and was amazed when it worked and his pain was relieved. The great, though somewhat perplexing, thing about sharing the spray with him was I needed only to refill the bottle with bottled water when it got low, and it was magically replenished. I still, to this day, don't understand it, but it works. I have used it on headaches and sore muscles, but really anything that is sore or hurting. My friends even borrow it to use for their arthritis; they call it liquid gold.

Facebook Entry October 20, 2014

> To those of you who know me well, I'm sure this is no surprise but... WOWZA, I may have overdone it a little today. Not sure whether I was trying to prove my improvement to myself or others. Comfy shoes may have helped [in the deception] too!

Chapter Forty

Shock Therapy Anyone?

On my first night back I performed a bacterial shock therapy, and I got up just three times during that night. I was encouraged enough that I turned off the Interstim. The bacterial shock consists of a mixture of wild harvested Devil's Claw, Echinacea and Olive leaf extract.

Remember back before we left, how Doug and I vowed to do whatever Jack said? One of his orders was to put up a sleep shield, though I could see Doug roll his eyes at the mention of such an oddity. We installed the sleep shield, though somewhat begrudgingly on Doug's part, and within a couple of days Doug was sleeping like a baby!

The sleep shield is used to ground the body to earth. A metal screen is placed between the mattress and box spring, as well as up against two of the bedroom walls. A copper wire is then run through them and to the ground plug in the wall. Also called earthing, grounding is based on the discovery that connecting to the Earth's natural energy is foundational for vibrant health. When we make direct contact with the surface of the Earth, our bodies receive a charge of energy that makes us feel better, fast.

Later that same week I was forced to turn the Interstim back on. I had hoped to be sleeping through the night by now and not have to wear pull-ups any more, but that wasn't my case.

Two weeks and one day after the treatment I seemed to have taken a few steps backward. My bladder was not good, my walking was not strong and everything required way more effort. I felt sad. And scared. His Word was again my go-to, and my hope.

And we know that in all things God works for the good of those who love him, who have been called according to his purpose. ~Romans 8:28 NIV

It was now time for me to do the fungal shock, which consisted of a mix of Essential Flora, FOS powder, Citricidal, and Candida Digest. Following the Fungal shock, I had the best night's sleep in years. I slept hard and was delighted to have only gotten up twice.

One-Month Update

Facebook Post November 10, 2014

One month ago today we left on a "hope for healing" adventure. Many of you prayed and continue to do so. So, I am writing tonight with my one-month update.

Before I left I used a cane and scooter at work. After a day's work I came home and sat on my butt, resting. Now, I will just tell you about my day today.

First I had hallway duty, prior to treatment was done sitting on my walker seat. This morning I did my duty, walking and using my cane.

I continued the rest of my Before I left [for Saint Augustine], my average nightly bathroom trips was eight to 10. This has improved greatly. I (we) now sleep SO much better! I've only been getting up one or two times a night. WOOHOO!!!

All I can say is PRAISE GOD!!! Thank you for your prayers. I'm not yet where I hope to be but he said it would take up to six months to reach full potential. I will still try to give updates periodically.

THANKS again for your love and support!

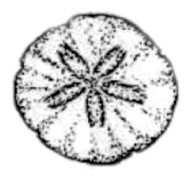

Chapter Forty-One

Doctor Goes AWOL

All of the issues seemed to fluctuate, so I was ready to talk to Jack and see what kind of recommendations he had. But for some reason, I wasn't able to reach him. His staff assured me that I was on his list to call, but all we got was silence. Frustration set in. I became highly concerned.

"Has the doctor called you yet?" my dad would ask every single day in a morning phone call.

I was glad that when we were there, Jack had explained the healing process to me and warned that there would likely be setbacks. I should expect to go through a time of rest before getting better. This helped, but I was ready to wrap up my two-month caffeine and mint fast. I just wanted to speak with him.

Chapter Forty-Two

New Doctor, New Diet

As November rolled around at school, we started a Biggest Loser Contest. I struggled to get started. I just couldn't seem to lose any weight, no matter how hard I tried. I added Weight Watchers to my plan and was working out hard each morning.

At this point I was back to doing my rider for 20 minutes each morning, along with some weight lifting, sit-ups and push-ups. I felt really good about working out again.

By Christmas I was down 15 pounds. Vegetable soup was a common staple; I made it by the large pot-full. Smoked salmon was another of my go-tos. Doug smoked the salmon and I made tacos with it several times a week. I drank nothing but water. I basically ate fish and vegetables, but it was working. I won the contest!

With Jack not responding to my efforts to contact him, I went on the hunt for someone in my area providing the same kind of service. In December I found Mark locally through a teacher at school, and I made an appointment to see him at his nutritional store. I was told it would be $85 for the visit and that he would do biofeedback. The appointment cost me over $200. His equipment was much more up-to-date than Jack's but seemed to do the same type of thing.

Mark wanted me to go on an extreme diet of no gluten, no dairy, fruit, sweets, pork or beef. What? I had already given up caffeine for the past three months! This left me fish, vegetables and water. He wanted me to buy 12 sessions for $850. I left feeling mad, sad, scared, less hopeful and discouraged. It would take me a couple weeks to figure out my next step.

In January I made the decision to see him once more. I took my notes and told him what my expectations would be should I purchase the twelve sessions. I wanted him to use the biofeedback and focus on my bladder—obviously still my first priority. Should he agree, I would then try the diet. Little did he know that I had previously given Doug a timeline of six weeks with Mark, and if no results by then, I'd be done. With Doug's blessing, I started the weekly appointments.

In January I started doing five flights of stairs each day with ankle weights on. I was getting stronger.

After the first six visits with Mark, I was feeling good but my bladder had shown no improvement. I had discussed the matter (of my bladder) with my MS doctor at my six-month checkup. I was hoping that his team would notice how well I was doing from the natural supplements, but they were indifferent. In fact, the doctor suggested that I get a catheter. Oh no, I was not giving up yet!

I went to Mark and told him how frustrated I was that after six treatments I had no improvements to show for them.

"I think you need to go see my mom," he said. "She does some different things, maybe she can help."

"Oh great; so now I'm supporting the whole family?" I thought.

"I don't want to see you again until after you see her." So, I felt I had no choice. At least her fees were very reasonable, compared to Mark's and Jack's. With an appointment on the books, I went to see "The Mom."

"I don't think it's your bladder," The Mom said, with magnifying glass in hand, peering into my eyes.

"I think it's your colon and your thyroid that are causing you problems, " she told me matter-of-factly.

"So, what should I do?"

"A 14-day colon cleanse," she insisted. So, I bought the cleanse and got started right away. What did I have to lose? I learned this type of procedure is called iridology. Skeptics call it quackery.

All I can say is Praise God! After the first week on the colon cleanse I had no more bladder issues. I seriously had no more bladder issues. None. I turned off the Interstim and was now getting up just a couple times a night. Oh my, I cannot express the relief and gratitude I felt. My entire being was in a constant state of thanksgiving to the heavenly Father. Thank you, precious Lord, for your faithfulness and kindness and answer to prayer. Thank you, God!

Up till now, my bladder issues were a secret known only by my husband and me. It is just such a humiliating and personal burden. But now, all of a sudden, I am telling the whole world how great my God is. God is amazing. God is great.

By March I was still off coffee but definitely ready to partake in the delectable treat once again. Resolving the colon issue came with its own struggles, but my bladder remained good. I continued to work on losing weight. Spring break was approaching, and I was nearing my goal weight.

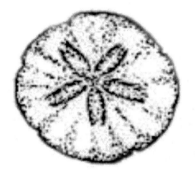

Chapter Forty-Three

Celebration

By the end of our spring, I had lost a total of 30 pounds in the Biggest Loser contest at work. I was finally at the weight my doctor wanted for me, and I was feeling much better about my appearance. I was especially glad that I hadn't gotten rid of my old clothes that had been too small. I may as well have had an all-new wardrobe since I hadn't worn my old clothes for some time, plus I didn't have to spend any money on new clothes—win/win!

Last summer I scheduled a spring break trip—a tropical paradise. Our once-in-a-lifetime trip would be our celebration. It was no longer our "spring break vacation" but now our "celebration vacation"

I've come so far in these past six months. We wanted to celebrate God's blessing and His healing. God surely knew back when I scheduled this trip that we would have something to celebrate.

Christine Ganger

Facebook Post May 9, 2015

> My grandson doesn't know it, but he just gave me the greatest Mother's Day gift. We were walking into church and he said "Hey, how come you can walk as fast as me now?" I could have cried! I love that boy and continue to thank God for His healing.
> Happy Mother's Day!

Chapter Forty-Four

Setbacks &
the Peace of God

J ust this past week someone at church asked me what I
think has helped me the most.

"Hope," I said after careful consideration. Having
hope after my doctor gave me none was the most help. It helped
me get up each day and work to move forward.

And that's how I thought I'd end this story—making it
about hope. But then I get this phone call from my principal. He
was going to be moving me back into the classroom.

He may as well have punched me in the gut. Knocked the
wind out of me. Just the thought of moving back to the
classroom exhausted me. Some in my situation would panic at
this news—or quit altogether.

After twenty years at this school and many friends later, I
was given the choice to go into the classroom, which meant a
torturous climb upstairs, or leave the building. I was mad, sad,
and scared, but I would do what was best for me. Knowing in
my heart that God had a plan and a purpose didn't prevent the
torrent of emotions that followed. This was an ambush; I never
saw it coming.

"We're not going to sleep tonight, are we?" Doug asked me as we lay in bed at the end of that deeply emotional day. Each emotion was like a wave crashing in on the one before it. I felt like I was drowning. My personal value was assaulted that day and I felt discarded, overwhelmed and of no use.

I have a routine that works for me in which I say the Lord's Prayer when I can't sleep. So I took a deep breath and began. I was beginning to feel a peace come over me when a Proverb came to my mind.

Trust in the LORD with all your heart, and lean not on your own understanding; In all your ways acknowledge Him, and He shall direct your paths.
-Proverbs 3:5-6 NKJV

I recited it silently as tears flowed. In my sadness blossomed this lovely peace; I could, after all, always trust God. None of this had been a surprise to Him. He has brought me this far, and I knew He would continue to guide and direct me just as He faithfully has in the past. Doug and I did, indeed, sleep that night. We rested well in the peace of the Lord.

Chapter Forty-Five

New Open Doors

I told my principal, that I wanted to be an interventionist and even asked—or insisted—that he call around town and find out what positions might be open for the coming year. Just as always, God already had things in place. A principal and friend I had done Summer School with in the past had an interventionist opening in her building. She welcomed me with warmth and kindness to her school.

That same day my principal sent an email to the staff letting them know of the change for the upcoming school year. The support and encouragement I received was overwhelming.

To give you a peek into how far I had come at this school, I'll share what it was like for those many years ago—20 to be exact. I had just remarried after my "scandalous" divorce, and my reputation branded me. I was an outcast in our building. I fully understood that it was the natural consequences of my actions, but I was determined to show my colleagues who I could be and who I indeed was already. I was determined to do my job and do it well. If others chose not to like me, that was their choice; but I would be professional. With each new year came new staff—people moved on either physically or emotionally. In time, I was able to establish myself as a good teacher and reliable friend and colleague.

This was one of the messages to me that brought me to tears:

"We will truly miss you! I can't tell you what your support and encouragement meant this year for my daughter and me as she continues her health struggle. So sad to see you go." ~TSM

Chapter Forty-Six

My Prayer for You

A snippet from my morning prayers before I head to work these days:

> Father, you've been so very good to me, and I give thanks for your blessings and for your faithfulness to me. Thank you, Lord, for a new day and the opportunities that lie before me.
>
> I would like to ask, Lord, that you would shine your light through me, making me a bright light for all of your lovely children with whom I come in contact today.
>
> Please be my strength throughout this day, and use and enable me to love and encourage others as only you can do.
>
> Thank you from the bottom of my heart for allowing me to hear the kindness and gratitude from their hearts toward me. It has been most uplifting and humbling and I love you for the gift.
>
> Thank you, Father, for answered prayers. And thank you for hope and a future

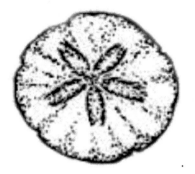

Conclusion

Today I have lived with Multiple Sclerosis for well over half my life. I believe God is, indeed, writing a story with my life, and I am humbled each day by that truth. With the effects MS has had on my body and with each trial I face, my faith continues to grow.

I have watched God work through each situation, and I am not angry or bitter because of it. In fact, I know that through it all, God has changed me. I am not who I was; but I believe because of the MS, I am becoming who God wants me to be.

I will continue to push and persevere in my weekday morning workouts. I know that this has helped strengthen my body and keeps me mobile. A couple years ago I would have never dreamed I would be able to do 20 minutes on the elliptical. Now, however, I do that three mornings a week before school, in addition to some weights, sit-ups and stairs. I am not giving up hope that one day God will allow me to run again. I know that would require strength and healing of my balance. God is so much bigger than any disease!

I pray daily that I can invest in Eternity. I hope and pray that, as a result of God's work in me, I can do that. I just want to love and encourage others. I want to offer hope and honor Jesus Christ.

To You, the Reader

I want to encourage you in whatever you are going through. No matter the outlook or diagnosis, always choose hope! Hope gives you the strength to get up in the morning and take the next step.

Please know, in the depth of your being, that you are never alone. The divine is with you. God wants to hold your hand and walk with you through each step.

If you're unsure of how to reach out to Him, it's as easy as closing your eyes, quieting your mind, and simply talking to Him. Because he has put His Spirit in you, it's just a matter of going inward and starting a conversation with Him. It is through regular prayer and contemplative quiet times like this that you will grow closer in communion with Him, and out of communion with the Great Divine comes peace, joy, and hope.

Father, I thank and praise you for the healing you have done and are yet to do.

May the God of hope fill you with all joy and peace as you trust in Him, so that you may overflow with hope by the power of the Holy Spirit.
~Romans 15:13 NIV

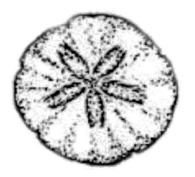

Connect with the Author

I would love to hear from you! If you were impacted in any way by this book, please shoot me an email and let me know. And if you want to share a piece of your own story with me, I would be delighted to hear it. If you have questions about what I've written or about the wonderful God I know, I would be happy to be a guide and friend to you in your search for knowledge.

Email me at: WalkOfhope104@gmail.com
Or find me on Facebook at: www.facebook.com/WalkofHope/

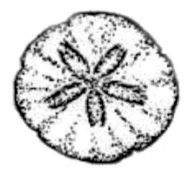

Epilogue

I pray that your *Walk of Hope* will bring you closer to both God and the healing you seek, whether spiritual, emotional or physical.

We go through many walks in our lives. I was blessed as my walk in earlier days brought me closer to God. I experienced His grace, mercy and love in spite of my poor choices.

As I continue in my journey, my *Walk of Hope* is:

- for God to continue the process of healing in my body
- for perseverance to continue my daily workouts, which in turn strengthen my legs and build endurance, and
- for people to see God through my actions and faith

What does your walk look like: long and tedious? Dismal? Or, have I helped you realize God does not give us more than we can handle and that He is with us every step of every trial on our walk?

May your Walk of Hope bring you closer to God, experiencing both peace of mind and heart.

CPSIA information can be obtained
at www.ICGtesting.com
Printed in the USA
FFOW04n2010061116
29073FF